ALL YOU WANTED TO KNOW ABOUT

Reiki

GW00640760

SUMEET SHARMA

New Dawn

NEW DAWN
a division of Sterling Publishers (P) Ltd.
A-59 Okhla Industrial Area, Phase-II, New Delhi-110020.
Tel: 26387070, 26386209; Fax: 91-11-26383788
E-mail: ghai@nde.vsnl.net.in
www.sterlingpublishers.com

Published by Sterling Publishers Pvt. Ltd., New Delhi-110020.
Lasertypeset by Vikas Compographics New Delhi-110020.
Printed at VMR, New Delhi.

*This book is dedicated to the
Lotus Feet of Bhagwan
Sri Sathya Sai Baba*

Contents

4

A Blessing from the Masters

May you have
Enough happiness to keep you sweet,
Enough trails to keep you strong,
Enough sorrow to keep you human,
Enough hope to keep you happy,
Enough failure to keep you humble,
Enough success to keep you eager,
Enough friends to give you comfort,
Enough wealth to meet your needs,
Enough enthusiasm to look forward,
Enough faith to banish depression,
Enough determination to make each
day better than yesterday.

Introduction

REIKI pronounced as RAY KEY is a natural system of hands in healing used since thousands of years. Reiki is a Japanese word comprising two parts — REI and KI, and these are Japanese Kangi characters.

REI means universal spiritual wisdom or consciousness. The wisdom that comes directly from GOD or the HIGHER SELF. It is not only God-conscious but is also all knowing. It understands each person completely, with the root cause of he

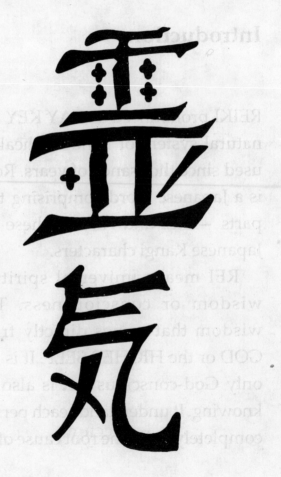

person's problems and difficulties, and knows how to heal them.

KI means the life force, and this is referred to by the Chinese as the CHI, by the Indians as PRANA and by the Hawaiians as MANA. Anything that is alive has a life force circulating and surrounding it, but the life force departs when it dies.

When the life force is high and free-flowing, one is less likely to get sick, and vice versa. It animates the body and is also the primary energy of our emotions, thoughts and spiritual life. KI is present all around us and can be accumulated and guided by the mind.

There is no doubt that Reiki energy is present everywhere. But one cannot learn Reiki healing by merely reading books because one has to be initiated as a Reiki channel or a healer by a Reiki Master. The attunement process is a sacred and secret one. It opens the psychic Chakras in the body, and establishes a spiritual link between the student/channel and the Reiki source.

Origin of Reiki

Reiki was rediscovered by a Japanese, *Dr. Mikao Usui* in the late 19th century. Hence Reiki has acquired the Japanese name.

Reiki is basically as old as the discovery of mankind itself. It was, however, in use for a long time without any distinct identity. Information from clairvoyants like Michelle Griffith throws light on the origin and metaphysics of Reiki.

According to Michelle, Reiki was originally brought to the earth by the GREAT BEINGS during the

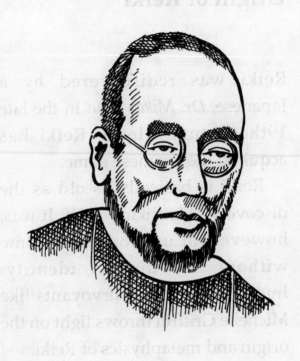

Lemurian times over 1,00,000 years back. This was the place where humans were first incarnated on the earth. They had a GREAT BEING amidst them who revealed the secret of Reiki.

Finally when LEMURIA sank, the knowledge of Reiki was also lost. The GREAT BEING also realised the problems emerging out of the negative Karma, viz., greed, lust, anger, jealousy and delusion. Reiki helped in overcoming these, and being a perfect energy established the connection with the GOD. Reiki does not expect one to be spiritually inclined for it to work, because Reiki is *UNCONDITIONAL HEALING ENERGY*.

Reiki was again brought back to the earth by the GREAT BEING to the Atlantis City some 50,000 years ago. People of the Atlantis believed in reasoning and were a direct opposite of the Lemurians. However, Atlantis also sank, and with it the treasure of Reiki energy.

Some 7,000 years back, during Egyptian Civilisation, Reiki was once again brought back for the third time, and continues to remain with us even today. Of late Reiki has made its presence felt in most of the countries

— India, the USA, Canada, Japan, Singapore, Europe, Australia. No one has complained of adverse effects of Reiki on them.

The clairvoyants of the New Age School of thought believe that Reiki is a contract between Mother Earth and God, in order to heal Mother Earth and the denizens. Moreover, Reiki is very simple to use. Reiki heals one physically, emotionally, mentally and spiritually, offering solutions to most known diseases and maintains the connection with god.

Rediscovery of Reiki

Dr. Mikoa Usui was the principal of Doshisha Christian University in Kyoto, Japan in the early 18th century. Once when he was asked by one of his students as to how Jesus Christ healed his followers, Dr. Usui could not give an answer to this question. Ashamed of not being able to answer, he resigned from his principalship and started his quest to discover how Christ healed.

He travelled to Chicago and studied there for seven years and acquired his degree in theology, although he was unsuccessful in finding the answer to his question. He later travelled to India and Tibet, learnt Sanskrit, and finally studied the sacred Tibetan Lotus Sutras and found clues to the healing power of Jesus. He then returned to Japan and focused on Buddha as he was known to have performed the same miracles as Jesus. Dr. Usui's journey finally led him to the Zen Monastery where he read the Sutras, writing and teachings of Buddha. On the advice of the monks he took to meditation.

Dr. Usui meditated for 21 days atop a holy mountain near Kyoto called "Kuri Yama". Fasting and continuously meditating for 21 days, he received enlightenment when a golden light hit his forehead with sacred Reiki symbols and he heard a divine voice.

The effect of this revelation was so strong that Dr. Usui woke up, but he did not feel the slightest exhaustion in spite of the prolonged fasting. Instead he felt fully energised. The feeling has been compared to the feeling of Archimedes when he said, "Eureka".

Dr. Usui ran down the hill in excitement and hurt his toe, and it started bleeding profusely. Dr. Usui placed his hands on the area of pain and the pain vanished in minutes.

Since he was feeling very hungry, he headed for the nearest eating place, and ate beyond his capacity. The surprised owner of the restaurant even advised Dr. Usui against eating too much after having fasted for so many days. But since Dr. Usui was empowered with the Reiki energy, no side effects whatsoever were observed.

He went to the Zen monastery the following day, and on seeing a monk suffering from acute arthritic pain, he simply placed his hands on the area of discomfort, and the monk was relieved of the pain.

These were the three miraculous experiences in the life of Dr. Usui which he had on rediscovering the Reiki power.

Dr. Usui continued his healing at the "Beggar's kingdom" near Tokyo and started giving free help to all. He found that they had no gratitude for his efforts.

He realised that in any action of man or in teaching there should be an exchange of energy, thus Karmically releasing the other person from any debt that may take fruit in the future. 20

Dr. Usui released his five spiritual Principles of Reiki detailed below:

Just for today, I will let go of anger.

Just for today, I will let go of worry.

Today, I will count my many blessings.

Today, I will do my work honestly.

Today, I will be kind to every living creature.

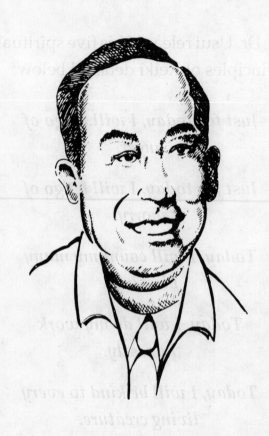

Dr. Chujiro Hayashi

Dr. Usui continued to teach throughout the island of Japan till 1926. During this period he had gathered 16 teachers. One of them was *Dr. Chujiro Hayashi*, who founded the first Reiki clinic in Tokyo. One of Dr. Hayashi's favourite students was *Mrs. Hawayo Takata*. She was born in the Hawaii Islands. She became a widow at a very early age and suffered from many ailments. When she met Dr. Hayashi, her normal health rapidly returned due to Reiki and she succeeded as a grand master in 1941. Before her demise on 11th December, 1980, she had already created 22 Reiki Masters in the USA and Canada.

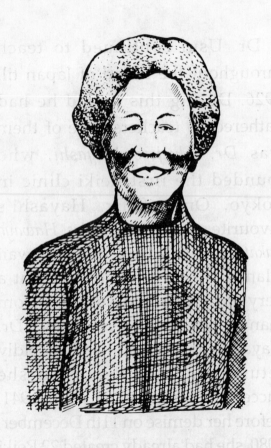

Mrs. Hawayo Takata

Today, Reiki is represented by three organisations; two of which are in the USA and the third is in Europe. They are namely:

- *The America International Association of Reiki*

- *The Reiki Alliance*

- *The International Association of Reiki which has its offices in Scotland, Poland and the Czech Republic*

The best part of Reiki is that it crystallises very well with any therapy be it the conventional Allopathy, Ayurveda, Acupressure,

Chiropractic, Aromatherapy, Shiatsu, Bach flower, Homeopathy, Massage, Yoga, Meditation and even Hypnosis.

Characteristics of Reiki Energy

Reiki is a spiritually guided life force energy because the God-consciousness called *Rei* guides the life force called *ki*, and these two jointly become *Reiki.* All those who use Reiki can practically experience how it guides itself with its own wisdom. The Reiki energy automatically flows to heal wherever the healing is required, although the practitioner may have overlooked the exact area where healing is required.

It has been observed by the clairvoyant that Reiki energy is bipolar in nature. It is made up of both male and female healing energies. The male part comes from above, i.e. the crown and other higher Chakras and is known as the *Shiva* energy in the *Tantra Yoga* and the female part comes from below, i.e. Root Chakra and is known as the *Shakti* energy in the *Tantra* system. These two energies communicate with each other and decide how much of each polarity is needed so that when the energies leave the hands they have the proper combinations of male and female healing energies.

One would be amazed to note that when more than one person works on a subject, the Reiki communicates with all the practitioners involved, channelling the male energy from some of the practitioners and the female energy from others, and properly mixing the two energies needed to heal the subject.

Reiki can never cause harm as it is guided by the God-consciousness. It always knows what a healee needs and adjusts itself to create what is appropriate for the person. One need not worry about whether to give Reiki or not because it is always helpful.

Moreover, since the practitioner does not direct the healing, nor decides what to work on or what to heal, because he is only a channel or an instrument through whom the Reiki or the universal life force energy flows to the healee. The healer is also not in danger of taking on the Karma of the subject being treated. It is not the practitioner who is doing, the healing so there is no room for the ego of the practitioner to come in the way of the free flow of the energy of God.

Reiki practitioners' energies are never depleted as it is a channelled healing. The practitioner continuously receives the universal life force energy once he or she is attuned. Reiki consciousness considers both the practitioners and the subject requiring the healing; so both get treated/healed.

Reiki is slow but positive energy. Reiki always increases one's energy and leaves one surrounded with a feeling of well-being.

Psychic Chakras in the Body

Psychic Chakras as shown in the figures are gateways of energy and life in the physical body. Each Chakra is associated with the glands and organs of the body. They react and respond to the energy and vibration received from Reiki, Yoga, Music, Colour, Acupressure, etc. Imbalance or stress arising due to the emotional, mental and spiritual state of an individual brings about disharmony of energy flow in the Chakras, resulting in physical illness.

Details of the Chakras

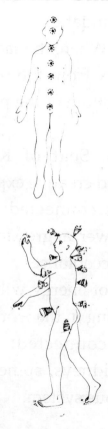

1. **Root Chakra (MOOLADHARA)** means foundation.

Location: Where the sacrum joins the coccyx from the rear to the middle bottom of the pubic bone in front.

Function: Seat of Kundalini energy and creative expression.

Emotions connected: Survival issues, power, aggression, vitality and self-acceptance.

Blockage of energy will result in fear of being in the world.

Organs connected: Adrenal glands, kidneys, spine, bladder and nervous system.

Diseases: Ailments of legs, hips and buttocks.

Ruling planet: Mars (solar, masculine).

Colour associated: Red.

Sounds associated : *Vang, Shang, Kshag* and *Sang*.

2. **Sacral Chakra (SVADHISTANA)** means the dwelling place of the self.

Location: Below the navel above the pubic bone.

Function: Sexual energy, feelings and emotions.

Emotions connected: Sexuality, sensuality, sensitivity, creativity, family bondage and social behaviour.

Blockage of energy will result in lack of self-acceptance, self-love and ego.

Organs connected: Ovaries and testes, fluids in the body.

Diseases: Bowel and bladder problems, irregular menstruation, premenstrual syndrome, impotence in both sexes, and disorders in the reproductive system.

Ruling planet: Mercury (lunar, feminine).

Colour associated: Orange.

Sounds associated: *Bang, Bhang, Mang, Yang, Rang* and *Lang*.

3. **Solar Plexus (MANI PURA)** means the city of gems, and is also the center of power.

Location: Above the navel and below the rib-cage.

Function: Centre of power and wisdom.

Emotions connected: Attachment to people and things, and relief from stress and gut feeling.

Blockage of energy will result in fears or anxieties about external things.

Organs connected: Stomach, adrenals, liver, gall bladder and digestive system.

Diseases: Cancer, arthritis, constipation, ulcer, migraine and heart diseases.

Ruling planet: Sun (solar, masculine).

Colour associated: Yellow (inspiration).

Sounds associated: *Dang, Dhang, Rlang, Tang, Thang, Pang* and *Phang.*

4. **Heart Chakra (ANAHATA)** means unstriken.

Location: Center of the chest, or sternum.

Function: Compassion, and love.

Emotions connected: Humility, tolerance, empathy, responsibility, unconditional love, healing center and spiritual thinking directly connected to the soul.

Blockage of energy will result in lack of emotion, security and fear of communicating with strangers because of past bad events

Organs connected: Thymus gland, heart, blood pressure, blood circulation, lungs and immunity centres.

Diseases: Heart diseases, blood pressure, disorder of the circulatory system, and diseases connected with the immune system.

Ruling planet: Venus (lunar, feminine).

Colours associated: Green and pink.

Sounds associated: *Kang, Khang, Gang, Jang, Jhang, Tang.*

5. **Throat Chakra (VISHUDDHA)** means pure.

Location: Throat.

Function: Communication.

Emotions connected: Self-expression, individuality, peace loving, creativity and trust.

Blockage of energy will result rigidity and frustration, specially in communication.

Organs connected: Thyroid gland, oesophagus, voice box, lower jaw and neck area.

Diseases: Problems related to the throat and lungs.

Ruling planet: Jupiter (masculine).

Colour associated: Bright blue.

Sounds associated: *Ang, Aung, Ahang* and *Ring*.

6. **Brow Chakra (AJNA)** means authority and unlimited power.

Location: Above the eyebrows in the centre.

Function: Intuitive power, will-power and clairvoyance.

Emotions connected: Overall personality balance, ambition,

telepathy, assertiveness, capability to realise current plans as reality in future, creativity and artistic nature, gentleness and receptivity.

Blockage of energy will result in confusion in the above emotional plane.

Organs connected: Pituitary gland, endocrine system, nose, ears, sinuses, nervous system, hypothalamus and lower brain.

Diseases: Hormonal imbalance, headaches, migraines, dizziness, depression, ear and eye problems.

Ruling planet: Saturn (masculine).

Colour associated: Indigo blue.

Sounds associated: *Hang* and *Kshang*.

7. **Crown Chakra (SAHASRARA)** means thousand petals and also means *Shunya* (zero).

Location: Top of the head.

Function: connection to our higher or spiritual self.

Emotions connected: Unity with all things, inner feeling development, consciousness and transpersonal awareness.

Blockage of energy will result in loneliness.

Organs connected: Pineal gland.

Diseases: Psychotic disorders, severe grief, deep shock and inability to face reality.

Ruling planet: Ketu.

Colour associated: Violet, white and gold.

Sounds associated: *Ah to Ksha.*

In some yogic breathing exercises, the sounds of each chakra are used to vibrate those individual chakras. However, the common sound which resonates with all chakras is *Aum* which means *I am*, the first sound of the universe and not the Hindu mantra *Om*. The astronauts during their travel in space have also reported the *aum* sound in space and it is this sound which vibrates with our Chakras.

44

One can draw further inference from the striking balance of nature through the seven colours in the sun's rays (VIBGYOR) which are in turn connected to each of the seven Chakras. There are seven notes in music — SA, RE, GA, MA, PA, DHA, NI, or DO, RE, ME, FA, SO, LA, TE and also seven days in a week. In other words, there are only 7 medicines for all ailments. Indian classical music is also famous for *Ragas* and *Raginis* made from the seven notes of music. This only goes to prove the deep understanding of the human body by our ancestors, who composed soothing melodies for every occasion from morning to night to create the right mood and atmosphere.

In Hinduism, there is a practice of worshipping different deities on different days of the week, viz., Lord Shiva is prayed to on Mondays as the *Shiva* energy is highest on Mondays, and this *God* or *Energy* on Monday is sure to be manifested into reality.

Aura

The invisible double of our physical body is Aura. This etheric body is made up of the fourth state of matter known as bio-plasma, and it exists around us. Since the vibrations are at a higher frequency, the human eye cannot see its existence. The Aura contains the exact blueprint upon which the physical body is shaped and anchored. It contains the structure that allows us to absorb high frequency energy of various kinds, including the vital life force energy, Prana.

Prana is absorbed into the physical body through the energy centres called the Chakras. These chakras facilitate the flowing in and out of energy. The chakras also distribute Prana and control and energise organs. They are also responsible for psychic activation.

Aura has seven layers corresponding to seven colours or VIBGYOR, (Violet, Indigo, Blue, Green, Yellow, Orange, Red). The red Aura connected to the base or Root chakra is the closest to the physical body than the others. Auras overlap each other one by one and the last is the spiritual Aura corresponding to the violet colour.

Picture of Aura

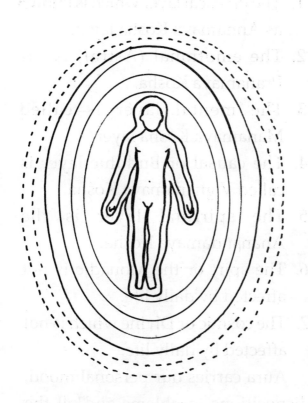

The seven layers or sheaths are:

1. The physical layer which is known as Annamaya Kosha layer.

2. The emotional (Astral) is the Pranamaya Kosha.

3. The mental layer is called Manamaya Kosha layer.

4. The causal or Buddhic layer is called Vignanamaya Kosha.

5. The spiritual layer is the Ananandamaya Kosha.

6. The spirt or the Monadic is not affected by daily life.

7. The cosmic or Divine which is not affected by daily life.

Aura carries our personal mood, dispositions, problems and all the experiences of life. When we hold another being's energy, opinion, consideration or judgement in our Aura, we create a block. This resistance comes in the way of developing our highest psychic potential. Hence we should hold our energy within our Aura.

Characteristics of Aura:
- Each aura has its own frequency.
- Each aura interacts with the aural fields of others.
- The human energy field also interacts with animals, plants, minerals and other energy fields.

- The longer and more intimate the contact, the more is the energy exchange.
- Changes in the aura affects the physical, mental, emotional and spiritual aspects, and vice versa.

The bio-plasmic body is a mould for the physical body to maintain the shape, form and features despite years of continuous metabolism. They both are closely related. Anything going wrong with the invisible body affects the visible body and vice versa. The aural body with the help of chakras is responsible for the functioning of all systems like the endocrine, respiratory, digestive, nervous, urinary and reproductive systems. It also acts as a protective shield against germs and diseased bio-plasma. All toxins, wastes and germs are expelled by health rays perpendicular to the body through pores, thus purifying the whole body.

Causes of Diseases

A state of restlessness is a disease. Disease can be purely due to internal or external reasons or both. Our own emotions, fears, negative thoughts and mental attitudes are the internal reasons that result in a host of phychosomatic disorders, viz:

- Allergies and Sinusitis
- Eczema, hives
- Obesity and constipation
- Lack of appetite
- Haemorrhoids
- Peptic ulcer

- Asthma
- Blood pressure
- Bed wetting
- Migraine
- Alcoholism
- Hiccups
- Drug addiction
- Impotence
- Premature ejaculation
- Retarded ejaculation
- Vaginitis
- Infertility
- Frigidity
- Menstrual Cramps

Some of the problems caused due to wrong emotions are:

Accidents	:	Expression of anger, frustration and rebellious nature.
Asthma	:	Guilt and inferiority complex.
Arthritis	:	Perfectionist and self-criticism.
Cancer	:	Deep resentment, self-pity, hopelessness and helplessness.
Ulcers	:	Fear, high ego and lack of self-worth.
Migraine	:	Anger, frustration and over perfectionism.
Over-weight	:	Feeling of insecurity.

Pain	: Self-guilt.
Stomach upset	: Inability to digest ideas or experiences.
Tumour	: Not allowing healing to take place.
Swelling	: Bottled up feelings and tears.
Sinusitis	: Irritated by some one near.
Stiffness	: Inflexibility and resistance to change.
Skin Problems	: Threatened individuality due to others having power over you.

Each chakra emits its own aura.

a) Mooladhara (Root/Base) Chakra is connected to the Physical aura or 1st plane.

b) Svadhistana (Hara) Chakra is connected to the Emotional aura or 2nd plane.

c) Mani Pura (Solar Plexus) Chakra is connected to the Mental aura or 3rd plane.

d) Anahata (Heart) Chakra is connected to the Buddhi/Causal aura or 4th plane.

e) Vishudha (Throat) Chakra is connected to the Spiritual (Soul) aura or 5th plane.

f) Ajna (Brow/Third Eye) Chakra is connected to the Monadic aura or 6th plane.

g) Sahasrara (Crown) Chakra to the Cosmic (Divine) or 7th plane.

Let us take an example of how disease manifests itself in our body by our own thoughts.

a) A person thinks he is superior to others - this blocks celestial love coming from the 7th plane, and hence it results in a tear in that aura.

b) Some person's love being superior to that others will result in weakness of the spiritual aura

c) The person will behave in a superior manner, resulting in blocks and stagnated energy on causal aura.

d) The mental aura responds by making the person feel that he or she is superior.

e) On the emotional plane, it affects him by creating a doubt about himself whether he is superior or inferior. This results in two opposite forces in a constant conflict of "Can I?" "I cannot".

f) On the physical level, it causes fear, which is unreal, blocking off the last chakra from a free flow of

60

energy. This results in physical illness like ulcer, etc.

Thus any imbalance in the higher auras are progressively transmitted down to lower bodies, eventually causing physical illness. An athlete or a gymnast may have a good physical aura but his emotional and mental aura may not be so good.

Our Vedic system has also repeatedly insisted that a person be humble and devoid of ego. They had recognised this fact even 5000 years ago. This is also evident because of the fact that the average age of people was a 100 years and above in those days, but in the cyber age it has reduced to less than 50 percent.

The Kirlian camera developed by Dr Kirlian from Russia is able to give colours and images of the aura of any object whether living or non-living. Human aura is very sensitive and changes very rapidly due to external factors like stress, pollution, weather and our own emotions like anger, fear, sensuality etc.

The amazing fact about the photograph of a torn leaf taken by a Kirlian camera showed the aura of a complete leaf and not the tear whereas when seen through the naked eye, the physical appearance of the leaf is two separate pieces.

Hence, it should be possible to grow the cut portion of the leaf back as it exists in the energy field. So logically speaking, people who have lost limbs should be able to grow them back.

This field has attracted many scientists all over the world and considerable research is going on in this subject.

The external reasons could be consuming contaminated food, water or toxin that directly attack the critical working ograns such as the stomach, liver, lungs etc.

Diseases may also be due to our own aura being weak and when any external infections like the cold virus or the influenza virus attack us, we fall sick. It is very essential that we keep our aura strong and healthy by regular meditation, physical exercises, positive attitudes and spiritual connections. Our aura weakens when we have.

1. Wrong emotions.
2. Poor nutritious food.
3. Alcohol and other addictions.
4. Drugs.
5. Tobacco.
6. Lack of exercise.

7. Lack of fresh air.

8. Lack of rest.

9. Stress.

10. Negative habits.

11. No spiritual activity.

Disease may also be due to karmic reasons which has nothing to do with our physical health but is purely due to our deeds. Lots of people are confused about Karma which some interpret as the revenge of God. However, this is not true.

The universe works in perfect balance and every action has an equal and opposite reaction This is well proved by Newton's law. We are all

Picture of Weak and strong Auric Emanations

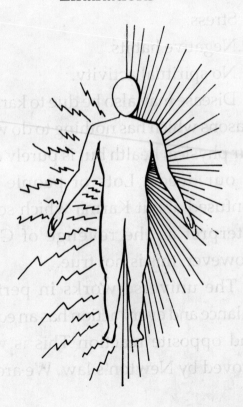

doing Karma consultant by physical actions, deeds, and thoughts, and these could be either positive or negative.

There is no doubt that all good Karma will breed good results and that all bad deeds would never give good reactions. This is the LAW OF THE UNIVERSE; well proved in the history of the world as well.

Constant resentment against self or others results in sickness due to our own fault. To neutralise the effect of negative Karma, the only way is to do positive Karma; if one tree is cut then plant two to compensate the negative action. It is very important to give to charity, do good deeds everyday and cultivate good thoughts. And to escape the negative thoughts that come to our mind simply say 'cancel, cancel, cancel' three times.

All positive and negative thoughts are very subtle energy produced by our mind which stays in our aura, and when constant thinking about the thoughts take place, there is an increase in the strength of these thoughts. Finally as LIKE ATTRACTS LIKE, we will have only those experiences which we have attracted which may be positive or negative. If we think of negative thoughts we are bound to attack only situations that would bring out these negative thoughts. Hence it is essential that we have only positive mental attitudes so that we attract only positive people and situations in our life.

Reiki helps to a great extent in neutralising the negative Karmic field. When we keep adding fresh water to a glass of salt water, there would be a stage when there would be no more salt in the water glass. The constant practise of Reiki would help one to overcome the worst effect of Karma to a great extent. If we were to lose a limb due to karmic effect, we may suffer the lesser effect of say a fracture or any other less severe disease.

Some Causes of Illness and Wanting it to Stay

- Unresolved guilt, grief or anger following a tragedy can give rise to illness, viz, self-punishment.
- Stress and bitterness due to the long-term care of a now-deceased loved one can cause life threatening illness that would be felt as an escape from despair.
- Illness can provide an escape from unhappiness in one's atmosphere at home or place of work because one feels entangled in a hopeless situation.

- A disregarded plea for help or reunion with a spouse over an unwelcome divorce may lead to illness in the heart-broken partner.
- The illness of one family member can be a cause of dysfunctional family's needs. Families may unknowingly want to maintain the illness of a member. By doing so there is balance and happiness amongst members of the family.
- Illness can be a means of manipulating loved ones, even by allowing the ill person to be dependent and cared for, and thus keeping family members from leaving the home front.

- Illness can also be a source of punishment to those with whom we are angry including ourselves.
- Illness can help one to escape from boredom, loss of meaning and self-worth. The examples of such illness would be the abandoning of home by children, retirement, conditions prevailing in poverty and unemployment.
- A distorted or faulty picture embedded in one's mind can lead to the belief that illness and death would visit one at a particular age as similar thing had happened to another family-member.

When one can recognise oneself in these situations one can escape illness and death as well by choosing life. One's present is often due to one's choice and one is fully responsible for one's own health and life. Therefore, one should believe in one's own ability to influence the circumstances in one's life.

Stages in Reiki Attunements

First Degree Attunement: This is the most basic Reiki degree in which the heart, throat, agna and crown chakras are initiated to enable Reiki energy to flow through the palms of the first degree holder. For first degree channels, the area of focus is on healing at the causal or physical level for one self and others. The specific healing positions, 28 in number, given by various Masters are taught. It balances the body emotionally, physically, mentally and spiritually.

After attunement, some students complain of discomfort like letting out of pent up feelings, severe headaches, vomiting, stomach upset, nausea, etc., which are considered to be good signs, as negativity of years within one's body finds a way of release. Hence, a 21-day cleansing period is prescribed by traditional *USi Masters* during which the receiver practises Reiki without fail, to drive out the negative energies in the body which may manifest itself in the form of physical disease.

Discomfort is not a necessary out come, and this does not mean that attunement is incomplete or that the person has not become a Reiki channel. However, complete faith and surrendering to Reiki is advisable for the II degree.

Second Degree: Three important symbols passed on by the Reiki Masters are taught to the II degree Reiki channels. II degree Reiki channels can even send distant Reiki to anyone anywhere in the world in addition to physical touch. The prime emphasis is adjusting the ethereal rather than the physical body and it is said that the vibration levels are four fold more in the II degree than in the I degree.

The II degree channels can send Reiki to past or future events in order to realise a goal or forget a traumatic event and cancel it from one's memory once and for all. It is recommended that Reiki II should be taken 21 days after the first degree to allow the cleansing period to be completed. The idea of going through the attunement process of the I and II degree on subsequent days are not acceptable to some of the traditional Reiki Masters.

The three symbols taught to the II degree channels are CHO-KU-REI (Power Symbol), SEI HEI KI (Emotional and Mental Healing

Symbols) and HON SHA ZE SHO NEM (Distant Healing Symbol).

Reiki symbols are transcendental in nature. They work at the subconscious mind and are directly connected to super consciousness. Whenever these symbols are used, "Rei" responds by changing the way the ruler energy function. This process has been created by a sacred agreement between the God and the Reiki channels. A person does not have to be in an altered state for symbols to work, as they work automatically. The symbols have their own consciousness which is explained in detail in the following pages.

Third Degree: III degree Reiki is divided into 3A and 3B. In 3A, an additional symbol of DAI-KO-MYO, the Master Symbol is given to open up the third eye and help in attaining personal growth, transformation and increased enlightenment. 3B is the Teacher's certification degree, for those who are keen to devote their lives to the art of healing, and further pursue their interest in the study of this universal life force. After becoming 3B, one can attune prospective Reiki channels of I, II, III

and A level. Additional Master
Teacher level is available to turn the
3A level into 3B.

Karuna Reiki

Origin of Karuna Reiki: Karuna Reiki was evolved by William L. Rand. The symbols were channelled by several Reiki Masters including Mercy Miller, Kellie-Ray Marine, Pat Courtney, Catherine Mills Bellamount, and Marla Abraham. William used the symbols and found them to have value, but felt that they had more potential than what was being accessed. He meditated on them and was guided to develop the attunement process and called the new system Karuna Reiki. Some of the symbols used in Karuna Reiki are used in other systems too, but they do not have the same effectiveness of healing energies as in the Karuna System.

Karuna Reiki is different from Usui Reiki and most of the channels find it equally powerful as the Usui Reiki. This energy has a more definite feeling and works at all the energy levels at the same time. Channels have reported that divine energy surrounds them and those who are being healed also feel it. Those receiving Karuna attunement experience their guides, angels and higher self, and the healing presence of the enlightened people.

Karuna is a Sanskrit word used in Hinduism, Buddhism and Zen. It basically means compassionate action, i.e. action that reduces the suffering of others. The Enlightened person views all beings as ONE and thus extends his Karuna to one and all, without any discrimination. When one helps others and aids them in their healing, the entire being is benefited. Compassionate action is not only extended to others out of love but because it becomes a logical action. It certainly makes sense to reliev all others who are in pain just as one would want one's own pain to be healed. Buddhism preaches that Karuna must be accompanied with prajna or wisdom for the right effect.

Karuna is the motivating quality of all enlightened persons who work towards ending the suffering of others. They continuously send the unlimited healing in addition to guiding us but we are not receptive to it. When one develops Karuna within oneself he or she is bound to help others and become more receptive to the Karuna that is being sent by the enlightened people. Thus Karuna Reiki opens one to work more closely with all the enlightened people whether present physically or in spirit.

While healing by touch or sending remote healing, the effect of the healing is much quicker and very powerful with karuna Reiki. However, Karuna has to be combined with Usi Reiki.because by itself, Karuna cannot be used to send distant Reiki. Karuna is made use of for diminishing specific problems. A few symbols have been given by Bhagwan Sri Sathya Sai baba too.

How does Reiki Heal?

Reiki energy being loving and powerful works at all levels, viz., physical, mental, emotional and spiritual, and to a great extent, even at the karmic level.

We are alive because of the life force flowing through us. Life force flows within the physical body through pathways called chakras, meridians and nadis. It is also around us in a field of energy called Aura. Life force nourishes the organs and cells of the body, supporting them in their vital functions. When this flow of life force is disrupted, it causes diminished function in one or more of the organs and tissues of the physical body.

The life force is responsive to thoughts and feelings. It becomes disrupted when we accept negative thoughts or feelings about ourselves either consciously or unconsciously. These negative thoughts and feelings attach themselves to the energy field and cause a disruption in the flow of life force. This diminishes the vital function of the organs and cells of the physical body.

Reiki heals by flowing through the affected parts of the energy field and charging them with positive energy. It raises the vibration level of the energy field in and around the physical body where the negative thoughts and feeling are attached. This causes the negative energy to break apart and fall away. In doing so Reiki clears, straightens and heals the energy pathways thus allowing the life force to flow in a healthy and natural way.

Points of Healing

Traditional Usui Reiki masters teach 26 points of healing in our body where we store different kinds of emotions and stress.

We store emotions related to different places as detailed below:

1. Nose : Sense of smell and sexual response.
2. Mouth : Capacity to take in new ideas.
3. Forehead: Intellectual expressions.
4. Neck : Stiffness due to with held statements.

5. Solar   : Power issues and
   Plexus   wisdom.
6. Genitals : Fear of life.
7. Knees   : Fear of death or ego
                or change.
8. Face   : Expressions to mark
                our personality.
9. Brow   : Intuitions.
10. Ear   : Capacity to hear.
11. Jaws   : Fear of expression
                and communication.
12. Chest   : Relationship issues,
                love.
13. Abdomen: Centre of sexuality,
                deepest emotions
                and feelings

14. Thighs : Trust in our own abilities and fear of inadequate strength.

15. Feet : Fear of completion and reaching our goals.

16. Hands : Fear of action and holding on reality.

17. Elbow : Strength of upper arms.

18. Upper Back : Stored anger.

19. Lower Back : Money and finance.

20. Ankles : Balance.

21. Arms : Connection in the external world.

22. Back   : Excess tension.
23. Ham-   : Self-control issues.
    strings
24. Lower leg : Fear of action.
25. Pelvis   : Survival needs.
26. Inner   : Sexually   charged
    thighs   issues.

Emotional Release Points

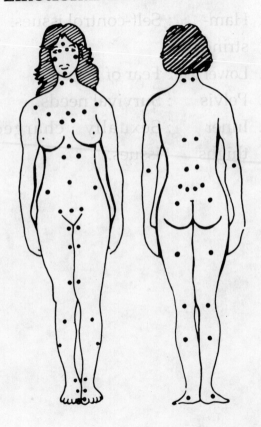

Attitude of Gratitude

It is very essential to acknowledge Reiki energy by saying the following "Attitude of Gratitude", before starting self-healing or healing the others.

"I thank the Reiki energy.

I thank myself for being here.

I thank (the name of the other person to be healed) for giving me a chance to give Reiki energy."

Hand Positions in Reiki

In the Reiki first degree, 28 points (7 major chakras and 21 minor chakras) are taught for self-healing as well as healing others primarily by way of physical touch on the area to be healed, for three to five minutes.

1. Eyes

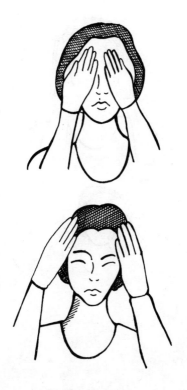

2. Temples

3. Ears

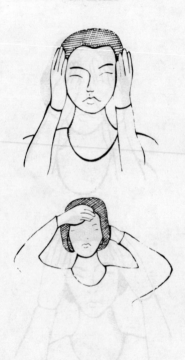

4. Forehead & back of the head

5. Both hands at the back of the head

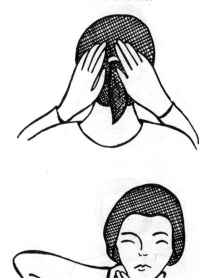

6. Throat chakra

7. Thymus & thyroid glands

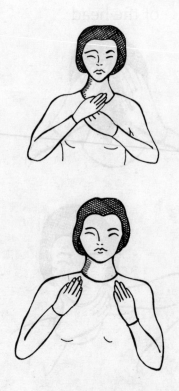

8. Lungs

9. Heart chakra

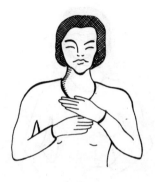

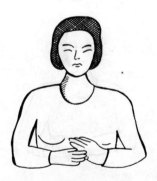

10. Solar plexus

11. Liver

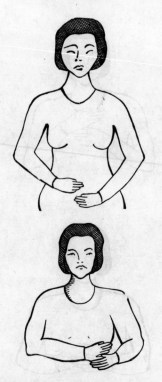

12. Pancreas and spleen

13. Hara

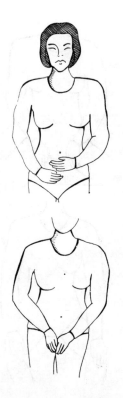

14. Root chakra

15. Thighs

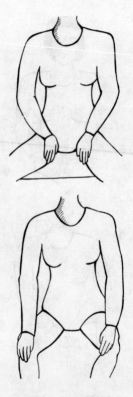

16. Knees

17. Calf muscles

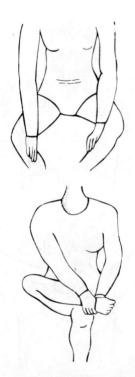

18 & 19. Ankles & soles
(left & right)

20. Shoulders

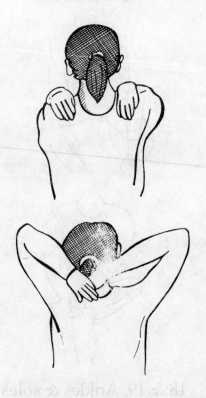

21. Thymus & thyroid glands

Guidelines On How To Treat Ailments With Reiki

Important points to note:

Reiki must be given to the chakras from both the sides.

The area requiring Reiki must always be treated along with the suggested chakras. Always study the medical report of the patient before administering Reiki. It is preferable to give full body Reiki treatment than partial treatment.

Problem	Areas to be Treated
Abdominal cramps	: Solar plexus chakra+ root chakra
Abscess	: Heart chakra + solar plexus
Acne	: All chakras
Addictions	: All chakras
Ageing problems	: Root chakra
Allergies	: Root chakra + throat chakra + third eye chakra
Anaemia	: Root chakra + solar plexus chakra + spleen chakra.

Anxiety	: Root chakra + crown chakra
Appendicitis	: Sacral + solar plexus
Loss of appetite	: Root chakra + heart chakra root chakra
Arthritis	: Knees chakra + soles of feet + solar plexus
Asthma	: Root chakra + throat chakra + third eye chakra
Back problems	: Whole spine + root chakra + solar plexus chakra
Bed wetting	: Knees + feet + root chakra + sacral chakra

Blood pressure (high & low)	:	Solar plexus + spleen chakra
Brain	:	Third eye chakra + back of head
Breasts	:	Solar plexus +sacral (cysts, lumps, + heart chakra soreness)
Breathing problems	:	Tips of lungs + heart chakra + throat chakra
Cancer	:	Root chakra + third eye chakra
Chronic Diseases	:	All chakras

Cold	: Heart chakra + throat chakra + eyes + ears
Constipation	: Root chakra + solar plexus chakra + liver chakra
Cysts, fibroid tumours	: Root chakra + sacral + solar plexus chakra
Deafness	: Heart chakra + solar plexus chakra + ears + temples
Diabetes	: Pancreas + solar plexus chakra
Ear problems	: Ears + heart chakra
Epilepsy	: All chakras
Eyes	: Eyes + heart + solar plexus chakras

Female problems	:	Heart chakra + sacral + root chakra + ovaries + throat chakra
General aches & pains	:	Heart chakra + root chakra + knees +feet
Headaches	:	Third eye + back of the head + whole spine + temples chakras
Heart problems	:	Heart chakra + solar plexus + root chakras
Hepatitis	:	Kidneys + all chakras + liver
Herpes	:	Sacral + solar plexus + third eye + crown chakras.

Impotence	: Root + base of spine + knees + sacral chakras.
Indigestion	: Sacral + solar plexus
Influenza	: All chakras
Insanity	: Crown chakra + solar plexus + root + heart chakra
Insominia	: All head points + knees + root chakra
Jaundice	: Liver + solar plexus + kidneys
Joint Pains	: Area of pain + chakra closest to it
Kidney problems	: Kidneys + solar : Plexus chakras

Leukemia	:	Root + crown chakra
Liver problems	:	Liver + sacral chakra + knees chakras
Lung problems	:	Root + heart chakras + tips of lungs
Migraine	:	Headaches + third eye + back of the head + whole spine + hara chakras
Neck problems	:	Heart + solar plexus chakras + back of neck
Nervous breakdown	:	Heart + throat chakras
Overweight	:	Root + sacral + solar plexus chakras

Rheumatism	:	All head points + whole spine + root chakra
Rheumatoid arthritis	:	Solar Plexus + head chakra + whole spine
Sinus problems	:	Heart + throat + third eye chakra
Skin problems	:	The area of infection + Root chakra
Spine	:	Whole spine + head + root chakra
Sprains	:	Root + knees + area of sprain
Sterility	:	Third eye + throat + solar plexus + sacral chakras

Stomach problems	: Solar plexus + sacral chakras
Stroke	: Crown + third eye + root + solar plexus + feet chakras
Throat problems	: All Head points + tips of lungs
Thyroid	: Thyroid + heart chakra + neck + root chakras
Tumours	: Heart + root + solar plexus chakras
Ulcers	: Root + sacral + heart chakra + knees
Urinary infections	: Hara + Root + Solar : Plexus + heart chakra

Uterus problems	: Sacral + solar chakra
Venereal disease	: Sacral + solar plexus chakra

Who can benefit most?

Reiki is for everyone; it does not distinguish caste, creed, sex, religion, age, object, animals and even plants. Reiki does not expect anyone to be spiritual or religious minded. It will flow equally through all after being attuned by a Reiki master.

One of the most important principals of Reiki is the "Principal of Energy Exchange", which Dr Usui had laid down when he realised the importance of fixing a fee in exchange for initiation given to a Reiki channel.

Exchange of energy between the Master and student can take place by way of money, object or wish, but the corollary to this is what is most dearest to the Master.

The Master should not make Reiki a way of business and bargain about the fees at any cost. They can, however, give some extra time for receiving payment or arrange for a proxy, but should refrain from giving Reiki free without proper exchange of energy.

Reiki can be learnt by children above 5 years up to any age as it is very easy to practise once one gets attuned. Reiki neither requires any diet regulation nor a particular time, it just flows freely and lovingly through all channels, always healing gently and completely.

Reiki is very helpful to housewives, executives, old people, teachers, children, physicians, professionals, nurses and others. It is handy too in healing during post-operative care. Reiki can also be given to a foetus, fractured parts of the body (preferably after the application of the plaster), boils, burns, skin eruptions and infections. Research done on AIDS patients in

the USA have also shown remarkable
recovery rates and tests have shown
a decrease of infection in patients.

Unconventional uses of Reiki

Treating animals with Reiki

The principal of treatment will always be the same. Domestic animals such as horses, cows, pigs, cats and dogs should be treated by laying the hands on the areas where the animal likes to be stroked, like behind the ears, under the neck and also in the area of pain. The hands should also be placed on the important parts of the body, like the head, heart and lower back. Let your intuition guide you in this regard. In smaller animals cover the animal with your cupped hands and give Reiki to the whole body.

Reiki can also be given to animals whilst they are asleep and from a distance.

Treating plants with Reiki

Plants grow very strong and healthy with Reiki.

Trees can be given Reiki at the trunks or you can even hug it and give Reiki through your palms as well as your heart.

Potted plants thrive very well when Reiki is given to the roots by holding the pot between your palms. You can also cup your palms lightly touching the plant from the top.

Seedling and seeds can be held inside your cupped hands and given Reiki. For best results try talking to your plant as well as giving it Reiki.

Treating non-living things with Reiki

Food, medicines, first aid articles, clothes, electrical goods, cars, batteries, and in fact, anything that may come to your mind can be treated with Reiki. Treatment is to be given by placing your hands on any prominent part of the article you are using.

Small articles can be held in your palms, and large articles can be covered by placing the hands on strategic places that may seem important to its well-being. Use your discretion for this.

You can also visualise very large non-living things as being very small and place your palms over it and give Reiki e.g., the house or apartment building you are living in.

Reiki flows into everything so let your imagination run wild and make the best use of this divine gift.

Recent Findings in Reiki

Ms. Paula Horan is a psychologist, Reiki Master/practitioner for over a decade, and authoress of a couple of enlightening books on Reiki. It was Paula's efforts that has made Reiki very popular amongst us today. During her recent visit to India in May 98, she shared some of the recent findings with many Reiki practitioners and others. She revealed that the Reiki which we all practise today is only the first of the seven levels of tantric teaching. Dr. Richard

Blackwell has come across Reiki founder Dr. Mikao Usui's own notes. Although only a part of the original scrolls have been translated, Richard has gathered much valuable information from Dr. Usui's manuscripts which he got in 1993.

Some further divulgence about Dr. Usui has disclosed that the Doctor was neither a Christian nor a dean of a school. But being drawn to healing, Dr. Usui studied Japanese and Chinese medicine, and allopathy as well. One day in his early youth he had a powerful vision which he shared with his peer's Shingon

Buddhist father, who took the Doctor under his fold.

Tendai and Shingon Buddhism, founded in the seventh century in Japan, was brought to Japan by Shuichi and Kukai. These two were trained by two different Indian Buddhist Masters in China. According to Richard, Dr. Usui may have been an incarnation of Kukai. Dr. Usui came across an ancient script, " The Tantra of the Lightning Flash which Heals the Body and Illumines the Mind". This manuscript which was brought to Japan by Kukai was in ancient

Japanese with Chinese annotations. Sadly, there was no living teacher who knew the tantra. So Dr. Usui began to practise all by himself.

Dr. Usui, in another lifetime as Kukai would have already mastered the practices. He again received empowerment through fasting and mastered the practices. Reiki III known to us presently is only the first of seven-level tantric teachings. It seems Dr. Usui poured water empowered by this tantra on his hands before healing. Dr Usui wrote, 'Reiki heals indirectly by calming the mind and raising the life-force energy,' whereas in higher levels of tantra one gets to learn to heal directly.

Learning Reiki: by Choice not by Chance

"Infinite is the source of joy. There is no joy in the finite. Only in the infinite is the joy. Ask to know the infinite".

Chandoyya Upanishad 7.23

Reiki cannot be learnt by reading books or by practising what is mentioned in the book. Although it is always more apt to learn any art or skill through an experienced Master or Guru who passes on his or her wealth of knowledge. In the case of Reiki one surely needs to learn through a Master or Teacher because the channel can be initiated to Reiki energy only through a Master. The attunement ceremony can be performed only by a Reiki Master. There is no religious ritual involved during the attunement. The Master uses certain techniques to invoke the presence of the Reiki energy and all the Masters, Angels and Spiritual guides as well, so that the initiation is done under the supervision of these higher beings. The procedure of attunement takes about 20 minutes. On being initiated into Reiki one will be empowered throughout the lifetime, whether one wants to continue the practice or not. The energy would start flowing through the palms the moment the channel express the attitude of Gratitude. The flow of energy can be experienced as a sensation of warmth or a tingling or coldness, and in some, there may not be any sensation whatsoever. It all depends upon how sensitive one is to the body. The channels should regularly heal another person and experience how the healing takes place on another person. Every time the channel heals another person, he or she is also healed because the healer is channelling the energy through him or her and passes it on to the healee.

Reiki is not Faith
Reiki is not Belief
Reiki is not Mind Control
Reiki is not Religion
Reiki is not Psychic Healing
Reiki is simply a loving and healing energy available in abundance in the universe. There is no logical proof nor can the Reiki energy be physically seen or measured. One can only experience the healing effect it has upon the channel.

Reiki teaching is not governed by any foundation or institution. All the Masters or Teachers become independent teachers of Reiki, and pronounce their own teaching standards based on their knowledge. Reiki being loving and benevolent flows freely, irrespective of whether the Master has put in a genuine effort to train the channels, guiding the students thoroughly without withholding any vital facts or not. Being empowered with this superior healing energy it does not do any good for the Masters to adopt any short cut methods while teaching and attuning Reiki.

Masters should have practice of healing self and others for at least a few years. However, there is nothing as bad masters or in correct attunement. All attunements are successful whether it is initiation by an amateur master or an experienced one, because it is the higher intelligence or the Reiki energy which descends to ensure that the channels are attuned successfully.

Very few Reiki Masters cover anatomy and the deeper causes of diseases so that they can be prevented or treated.

To select a Master the prospective student must take the following steps:

• Personally meet the Master who should be devoid of any EGO.

• He should have been into Reiki healing and teaching for a minimum of 2-3 years.

• He should teach 1st degree in one half or 2 full days and not just in a few hours.

• He must do at least 2-4 attunements for the 1st degree and single one for the 2nd and a higher degrees.

- A Reiki master cannot call himself a Grand master. Reiki Masters are actually Reiki Teachers. To be referred to as a Grand master, the Master should have actually reached the status of Dr. Usui.

- A Reiki master should give a detailed manual to each student as part of reference material in addition to the practice cassette.

- Meditation should be a part of Reiki training and it is certainly not very healthy to charge extra fees for teaching meditation.

- The fees should not be very exorbitant. The students are advised against bargaining because the fees are charged depending on the kind of training imparted. If a student negotiates the fee, then he or she is at a greater loss than the Master. The student would be receiving only that much of energy transfer for which he has paid, and the balance goes back to the Universe. This is the basis of the 'Energy Exchange Principle'.

• A student is likely to reach the doorstep of only that Master from whom he or she is predetermined to receive the Reiki initiation. One gets a good Master depending also on good Karma in the past.

• It is definitely a must for all the students to undergo practical training on how to heal oneself and others by practising in the presence of the master.

In order to obtain optimum benefit, the students are required to keep up the Reiki practice on a permanent basis. However, it is a must to self-heal for 21 days after each attunement of I, II and III levels, because during these 21 days one would be going through cleansing and at times it could even be 'crisis cleansing'. One should also complete all the levels in a sequence. Although a minimum of a 21 day gap needs to be allowed between the I and II levels, and about a 6-8 month gap between the II and III levels, Mastership should be thought off only after 3 years of extensive Reiki practise. There is misconception that higher levels of learning would make a person very powerful. One can be a good healer even after doing level I provided the channel has developed a sincere interest in healing has developed unconditional love for everything around, and has also surrendered to the energy.

Mastership should be taken up by only those who wish to teach and dedicate their time and effort to energy healing. Earning a living out of teaching and healing would be an automatic thing the Master would be blessed with but one should not focus all attention to make earning through energy an obsession. Keeping one's ego away, the master should have an attitude of gratitude towards all the students who come to learn Reiki from him, and the Master should thank the Reiki energy for all the guidance. Reiki being slow and sure-footed gently balances the Master until a state of near perfect balance is reached at all layers. Reiki would repeatedly create situations, and ensure that the Master has worked out all that is lacking.

By and large one should enjoy practising Reiki at all levels and experience the subtle grace. Although for all practical purpose it is sufficient to be a II level channel as one becomes a powerful healer, because even a Master uses only the II level technique for healing, along with the additional 'symbols of the master

Reiki Power: Your Passport to Spirituality

"All penances are in vain so long as selfishness endures lusting after worldly or heavenly pleasure."

Lord Buddha

The most common question often asked is 'Why has Reiki become so *famous* of late?' Two of the most simple replies are - Reiki is totally unconditional and secondly it is very simple to practice.

Sri Sathya Sai Baba says, "Every good action brings you closer to God and every wrong action takes you away. You decide where you want to go."

Religion is the first step to God and acts like the scaffolding to a building under construction. The moment the building is ready there is no need for the scaffolding. Similarly, spirituality is taking a journey within us and analysing all our actions through the questioning process (Prathahara). The awareness of living close to our nature or even in tune with our nature or in the present would result in a state of bliss. This would also aid one in

145

perceiving God. Buddha has mentioned this in his Dhammapada. We must learn to live by the principle of *"Thy Will, Not my Will"*. Reiki is one such gentle and caring energy that helps one in transformation through grace, and guides one to reach a state of spirituality beyond religion and rituals. It works at all levels — physical, mental, emotional, spiritual, karmic and genetic levels — in its own mysterious way, beyond the range of human understanding. On becoming the first degree Reiki Channel one can:

• Heal oneself with the physical touch of healing.

- Balance and harmonise one's body.
- Heal others with the healing touch.
- Treat plants, animals, vegetables, food, medicine and many other living and non-living things (as mentioned in the earlier chapter).

On becoming the second degree Reiki Channel one can:

- Heal oneself by using the three powerful Reiki symbols.
- Heal others anywhere in the world by using Reiki symbols.
- Heal others with the physical healing touch along with the powerful symbols.

- Send long distance healing energy to anyone in the world by using symbols and affirmations.
- Manifest personal goals.
- Protect one's property, house, vehicles and other belongings.
- Protect oneself during travel.
- Protect oneself from psychic attacks or black magic.
- Heal relationships for self and others.
- Heal the mother earth and the denizens.
- Heal past trauma.
- Program future events.
- Develop Intuitive and clairvoyant abilities.

On becoming Master/Teacher one can:

• Teach Reiki and also give Reiki attunements from first Degree up to Mastership.

• Fine tune the energy level of self and empower oneself with Usui Master symbol.

• Help oneself in personal and spiritual growth.

• Help oneself to drop the EGO.

• Go beyond beliefs, values, and judgemental tendencies, and identify one's limitations.

Traditional Usui Reiki Masters teaches Third Degree as a Master or a Teacher Degree. Some Modern Reiki Masters or Practitioners have divided the Third Degree into 3A and 3B which is not in tune with the Usui system of natural healing. One should aspire to become a Reiki Master or Teacher only when one has strong will power, knack of teaching and presentation skills, so that the channels created by them are worthy of being called Reiki Channels. Their higher beings and masters, through the seat of powered intuition, guide Reiki masters. Further, if a Reiki master does not teach after taking up the mastership, it becomes a nonconformance of the Usui's method of natural healing.

Tips on Self-Healing

"Neither reading the Vedas nor making sacrifice to the Gods will cleanse a man who is not free from Ego"

Lord Buddha

Reiki helps to heal oneself at all levels and elevates the soul for spiritual growth. Thus we can be freed from the cycle of birth and death. The steps to ultimate Bliss or Nirvana are:

1. Faith
2. Generosity
3. Purity in Thoughts and actions

4. Forgiveness to those who have hurt you
5. Honesty in relationships and earning
6. Contentment with worldly desires
7. Humility
8. Selflessness which is 'less of Self'
9. Compassion to the less fortunate
10. Patience
11. Detachment
12. Non Judgemental
13. Service Mindedness
14. Love for all

The apex of the healing pyramid is LOVE, Reiki also advocates the same

— Unconditional Love. One becomes a loving, caring and sharing being.

In addition to Reiki practice and meditation, one needs to introspect deeply within oneself to allow the healing to reach every cell, molecule and electron of the body, so that one could emerge as a fully healed and evolved being. It is very essential that one takes every step to heal oneself thoroughly because unless one is healed it would not be possible to heal others, or for that matter even teach others. It would be highly beneficial to all those who wish to become healers to take a little time off to answer the questionnaire. This would accelerate the self-healing process and can become a major part of the self-cleansing exercise. It is a must, particularly for all those aspiring to become second degree channels and even higher-level energy channels. All the questions must be answered truthfully setting aside the ego. There is absolutely no requirement to discuss the answers with any one because one is taking a journey towards one's core shedding all the layers accumulated over the years. By jotting down the answers and analysing them, we throw out the garbage from our mind, and when this takes place, we are in a healthier position to view everything as it is, accepting them as they are, without any prejudices whatsoever.

Questionnaire for Self-Cleansing

1. What do you like to do as a hobby? List all the things you love to do apart from your profession. Have you achieved that already?
2. What do you hate to do and why?
3. List all the people who have hurt you in your life. Are you willing to forgive them?
4. What angers you most in life? List all the situations, people, objects etc.
5. What are you dreams, desires and hopes? Are you working towards

them? Do you curse or take it as a challenge?

6. Do you see beauty around you or do you see only filth? If so list them both separately.

7. List the people you love and state one good reason why you love them.

8. List your good and bad points and regularly review them.

9. What are your bad habits and present addictions? Do you want to free yourself from the clutches of these addictions, and if so which one?

10. Are your present diet, nutrition and daily exercise adequate? Do you check what you are eating?

11. Are you a vegetarian? Do you include fresh juices, fruits, and salads (including greens, raw vegetables) in your diet?

12. Are you oversensitive to people's remarks, comments and criticism? If so, list what hurts you most and accept it.

13. List all bad traumas and situations you have had so far in your life. List all broken relationships if any and the reasons for being broken, highlighting your faults.

14. Do you make occasional visits to gyms, health clubs or beauty saloons to pamper yourself? If not why?

15. Is money very important to you? On a scale of 1-10 how would you rate money for your needs keeping your greed at bay?

16. What is your attitude to sex? Do you feel that it is good or filthy? Do you openly discuss sex or would you consider sex as a taboo subject?

17. What spiritual beliefs and values have you developed?

18. What are the superstitions that hold you back? List them and try

to find logical reasoning to superstions.

19. Do you believe in GOD? If yes, Why? If no, Why?

20. What kind of service projects have you been involved with to serve society? Do you give to charity?

21. Do you regularly practice meditation, yoga or any other spiritual practices like singing bhajans with a group, etc.?

22. List the good things you have done for others. Do you expect anything in return from them? Are you ready to forget the good

done by you without expecting any kind of compensation?

23. What is God according to you? Where does God exist?

24. Have you done any harm to anyone consciously or subconsciously in the past? Are you guilty of it? Are you ready to release your guilt?

25. Are you jealous of your friends/relatives/others for possessing things, which you do not have? If so list all the items.

26. Are you haughty about something special you are gifted with, such as beauty, wealth,

property, strength, power, materialistic possessions, knowledge, etc.? If so are you working towards quenching it?

27. Do you have any friend, or relative in whom you are able to confide?

28. Do you have the habit of writing down your feelings, which you are unable to express to others?

Reiki and Other Therapies

Reiki gels well with all holistic and alternative therapies including modern medicine.

It is a myth that Reiki competes with modern medicine or with the ancient practice of yoga, meditation, and other forms of ancient medicine. Reiki works gently in transforming a person into a loving, caring and empathetic entity. This again becomes possible only when one is keeping up the self-healing on a daily basis. A brief detail of all other therapies are given below:

Yoga: Regular practice of Yogic Asanas and Pranayama helps one to maintain good physical health, fitness and even longevity of life and one's aura, and the energy field gets strengthened. Reiki practice does not interfere with Yoga. In fact, the higher koshas, like the Vignanamaya and the Anandamaya koshas, get easily balanced and aid the ascension process of the soul. A strict regime is to be followed by Yoga followers to achieve optimum benefit. One needs to wake up early in the morning to do certain Yogic exercises; one cannot partake of food prior to certain asanas and Pranayama exercises, and there are many disciplines to be followed on a daily basis. These preconditions put the practise of Yoga beyond the reach of every human being. If a set pattern is not followed, one cannot obtain satisfactory results. Reiki works at cellular and sub-atomic levels, so any mistakes during breathing exercises, or while practising postures are balanced by Reiki. Being deeper than

Yoga, Reiki combined with Yoga, further brings about a greater balance of body, mind and spirit.

Nutrition : We are what we eat. And so we need to come out of the vicious cycle of addictions to salt, tea, sugar, alcohol, drugs, meat etc. Complete healing is only possible by getting rid of addictions and changing over to a *Sattvic diet* or one that is beneficial for a particular ailment. Our body techencially requires 1Kcal per minute, which is 1,500 Kcal per day, to survive. However, we overstuff ourselves with a minimum of 3,000-

4,000 Kcal per day. Reiki helps to stop the craving for harmful foods and also helps us of removing the negative effects in food or beverages, and makes it tastier, healthier and more palatable. A healthy diet comprises of fruits, raw vegetables, sprouts, wheat grain, soya products and small portions of meat (chicken and fish). Beef and pork should be completely avoided.

Acupressure and Massage: For those who practise acupressure and different types of massage therapies, Reiki is an additional asset, since

Reiki basically flows out of the hands and the fingers of the healers. Along with the massage and acupressure the clients will receive Reiki too. Most massage clinics and beauty saloons also train their staff at least to the 1st degree Reiki.

Homeopathy: The Principle of homeopathy is "Like cures like" by treating the disease with the cause of the disease itself. It activates the healing process within us. Reiki, also activates inner healing by calming the mind. Homeopathic medicines could be energised with Reiki and patients who have learnt Reiki could also do the same, adding to the efficacy of the medicine for quicker results.

Allopathy: Modern medicine works on the opposite principle of alternative medicine, that is, symptomatic relief and suppression of the effect, whereas causes remains untouched. That does not mean that mankind can do without modern medicine. In fact, it is the combination of allopathy and natural sciences, which works wonders and helps people recover faster. The use of drugs prescribed by the physicians themselves is a matter of faith because the medicines are developed by the multinational companies after carefully carrying out experiments on rats and rabbits. The doctor may not have any idea of the chemical composition of the drug and its complexity. Hence multiple drugs are prescribed for a single ailment and generally the patients get relief from the symptoms and diseases. Medicines can also be energised with Reiki symbols and they work faster and deeper with no side effects at all on the human body. This is immensely helpful as modern medicine has very little answer to diseases like asthma, diabetes, migraine, blood pressure, and other stress related problems.

Hypnosis and Mind Control: Since Reiki basically works on the mind, anything that calms the mind will enable Reiki to go deeper. When one is not open and receptive, one closes his outer aura and no healing energy can enter without the subject's permission. In the hypnotic state, if Reiki is beamed with strong affirmations, the recovery is faster, and a general change of attitude takes place. Healing addictions, wrong habits, emotional problems, low self esteem and confidence is quicker when we combine Reiki with Hypnosis or NPL or Silva Mind Control Techniques. For more information please read my book **"Reiki and Hypnosis for success and self realisation"** which gives complete information on how to combine both these sciences.

Crystal Healing: Crystals are semi-precious gemstones that house the energy, or work as capacitors of energy, both positive and negative. They are capable of producing a mechanical movement known as piezoelectric effect used in the quartz watches. Since they store energies, they can be given Reiki, and can either be carried in our wallets or worn around the neck with a chain, or as a bracelet within our aura level to continuously emit Reiki throughout the day. Semi-precious stones like amethyst, coral, moonstone, tiger-eye, and blue and pink quartz can be for personal use.

While healing, seven-colour healing stones can be placed on the subjects' Chakras. They are as follows:

Crown	:	Quartz
Agna	:	Amethyst
Throat	:	Blue Quartz
Heart	:	Pink and Green Quartz
Solar	:	Yellow Quartz
Sacral	:	Orange Carnelian
Root	:	Blood Stone

The Reiki symbols are drawn and transferred into the Chakras to energise, open, and harmonise them. Hence, crystals are additional assets to Reiki channels and healers.

As noted above, Reiki gels with all therapies without affecting their efficacy, and only works as catalyst in accelerating the effect for quicker results, so that the body is brought back to harmony at the earliest.